NATURAL REMEDIES FOR EVERYDAY AILMENTS

Unlocking The Secrets Of Traditional Healing Wisdom

By

Dr. Francis Williams

Table of contents

Introduction

In this busy, modern world, the appeal of natural remedies is calling us back to the basics of health and wellbeing. Let us take you on a journey with our eBook, "Natural Remedies for Everyday Ailments," to explore the amazing power of nature to help us feel our best.

1.The Power of Natural Remedies

For centuries, people have looked to the Earth's resources to help them feel better and stay healthy. In this book, you'll learn about the amazing healing power of natural remedies. We are still uncovering the secrets of herbs, spices, and holistic practices that can help us heal and revitalize.

2. The Importance of Holistic Health

As we embark on this journey, we'll discover a wealth of knowledge in the following chapters:
- Chapter 1: Common Ailments and Their Natural Remedies
- Chapter 2: Immune System Boosters
- Chapter 3: Natural Pain Relief
- Chapter 4: Skin Care and Remedies
- Chapter 5: Stress Management and Mental Health
- Chapter 6: Home Remedies for Cold and Flu
- Chapter 7: Natural Remedies for Allergies

- Chapter 8: Holistic Wellness and Prevention

In each chapter, we'll explore the various ailments and the natural solutions that can bring relief and restoration. We'll look into the healing potential of herbs, essential oils, mindful practices, and lifestyle adjustments. By the end, you'll not only have practical remedies but also the tools to live a balanced and healthy life.

As we go through these pages, remember that the power to heal and thrive is within you, ready to be unlocked. Let's unlock the wisdom of natural remedies and embark on a path to vibrant wellbeing.

Chapter 1

Common Ailments and Their Natural Remedies

In our hectic lives, it's not uncommon to experience everyday ailments that can take a toll on our health. Thankfully, nature provides us with a variety of remedies to combat these issues. In this chapter, we'll look at natural solutions for some of the most common concerns:

A. Headaches and Migraines

Headaches and migraines can be incredibly debilitating, impacting our productivity and overall quality of life. Fortunately, you don't always have to rely on over-the-counter painkillers. Let's take a look at some natural remedies.

1. Herbal Teas and Essential Oils

Herbal teas are a great way to naturally soothe headache symptoms. Brew teas with ingredients like peppermint, chamomile, or ginger, as these herbs have anti-inflammatory and calming properties that can help reduce the intensity of headaches. Additionally, essential oils such as lavender, peppermint, and eucalyptus can be used in aromatherapy to provide relief. Dilute a few drops in a carrier oil and massage onto your temples or take a few deep breaths of the scent for a calming effect.

2. Acupressure Techniques

Acupressure is a great way to reduce pain and relax. If you're suffering from a headache, you can target the webbing between your thumb and index finger, as well as the base of your skull. Spend a few minutes massaging or applying pressure to these areas and you should feel the tension and pain start to ease.

B. Digestive Issues

Digestive unease is a frequent issue that can interfere with our daily routines. Fortunately, there are natural remedies that can provide relief without the need for medications.

1. Ginger and Peppermint Remedies

Ginger has been a go-to remedy for digestive issues for centuries. You can enjoy it as a tea or add it to your meals. Its anti-inflammatory and anti-nausea properties can help with indigestion and nausea. Another option for digestive relief is peppermint. Peppermint tea or capsules can help with bloating and gas. However, if you have acid reflux, be careful with peppermint as it can relax the lower esophageal sphincter.

2. Probiotics and Fermented Foods

Having a healthy gut is essential for proper digestion. Probiotic supplements and fermented foods such as yogurt, kefir, sauerkraut, and kimchi can help introduce beneficial bacteria into your digestive system, which can help to create a balanced gut microbiome. This can help to reduce the symptoms of irritable bowel syndrome (IBS) and other digestive problems.

C. Sleep Problems

Getting a good night's rest is essential for feeling your best. If you're having trouble sleeping, here are some natural solutions to try:

1. Chamomile and Valerian Root

Chamomile tea is well-known for its soothing effects. Have a cup before bedtime to help you relax and drift off to sleep. Valerian root, which can be taken as a supplement, can also be beneficial for those struggling with insomnia and can help to create a sense of tranquility.

2. Sleep Hygiene Tips

It's essential not only to use herbal remedies, but also to practice good sleep hygiene. Make sure your bedroom is dark, quiet, and cool, and limit screen time before bed. Additionally, try to stick to a consistent sleep schedule to help your body's internal clock.

These natural remedies can help with common issues such as headaches, digestive issues, and sleep problems. Holistic health is about more than just treating symptoms; it's about promoting overall wellbeing. In the upcoming chapters, we'll look at more natural solutions to various health concerns, so you can take control of your health and vitality.

Chapter 2

Immune System Boosters

Our body's natural defense against sickness and disease is our immune system. Keeping it in top shape is essential for our overall health and wellbeing. In this chapter, we'll look at some natural ways to strengthen your immune system and keep it functioning optimally.

1. Vitamin C and Immune Health

Vitamin C is often praised for its ability to support the immune system. This water-soluble vitamin is known for its antioxidant properties, which help protect cells from damage caused by free radicals. It also plays a key role in aiding the immune system by stimulating the production and activity of white blood cells.

Incorporating foods that are high in vitamin C into your diet is a great way to naturally strengthen your immune system. Citrus fruits such as oranges, grapefruits, and lemons are well-known sources, but you can also find it in berries, kiwis, broccoli, and bell peppers. Why not make a habit of having a fresh fruit salad or a glass of homemade citrus juice every day?

2. Echinacea and Other Herbal Immune Boosters

Echinacea, astragalus, elderberry, and garlic are all great herbs to add to your diet to help strengthen your immune system.

Echinacea is a well-known herb that is praised for its immune-strengthening properties. It contains compounds that can activate the immune system, making it more efficient in fighting off illnesses. During cold and flu season, Echinacea supplements, teas, and tinctures are easily accessible and can be taken as a preventative measure.

Other herbs that can help boost the immune system are astragalus, elderberry, and garlic. Astragalus has been used in Chinese medicine for centuries to increase immunity. Elderberry is full of antioxidants and has been proven to reduce the intensity and length of cold and flu symptoms. Garlic has allicin, a compound with antimicrobial properties.

Echinacea, astragalus, elderberry, and garlic
are all great herbs to add to your diet to help
strengthen your immune system.

3. Lifestyle Habits for a Strong Immune System

In addition to taking dietary supplements,
certain lifestyle choices can have a major
impact on having a strong immune system.

- **Regular Exercise**

Doing regular exercise can help boost your
immune system by improving blood flow
and reducing inflammation.

- **Adequate Sleep**

Getting a good night's sleep is essential for
your body to rest, repair, and recharge.
Make sure you get between 7-9 hours of

sleep each night to ensure you are getting the quality rest you need.

- **Stress Management**

It's important to remember that chronic stress can have a negative effect on your immune system. To help reduce stress, try incorporating activities like meditation, yoga, or deep-breathing exercises into your daily routine.

- **Hydration**

It is important to stay hydrated for your overall health and immune system. Make sure to drink lots of water throughout the day.

- **Balanced Diet**

Eating a variety of fruits, vegetables, whole grains, and lean proteins is essential for providing your immune system with the nutrients it needs to stay strong.

Incorporating these immune-boosting strategies into your daily life can help to protect your body's natural defenses. It's important to remember that a holistic approach to health, which includes a balanced diet, herbal remedies, and healthy lifestyle choices, is the best way to keep your immune system functioning optimally. In the upcoming chapters, we'll look at more natural remedies for common ailments and continue our journey towards holistic wellbeing.

Chapter 3

Natural Pain Relief

Pain is something that all of us have experienced at some point in our lives, and it is essential to find ways to manage it in order to maintain our wellbeing. In this chapter, we will look at natural remedies that can help reduce pain and make life more enjoyable.

1. Arnica and Arnica-Based Creams

Arnica has been used in traditional medicine for centuries to help with pain and inflammation. Many people use arnica-based creams, gels, or ointments to soothe muscle aches, joint pain, and bruising. It is believed that the active compounds in arnica can reduce swelling and improve circulation to the affected area. It is important to follow the manufacturer's instructions when using arnica-based products, and to avoid applying it to broken skin or open wounds. If you experience any adverse reactions, discontinue use.

2. Turmeric and Ginger for Inflammation

Turmeric and ginger are two powerful anti-inflammatory herbs that have been used for centuries to help reduce pain, including arthritis and muscle aches.

- **Turmeric**

Turmeric contains a powerful compound called curcumin, which has strong anti-inflammatory and antioxidant properties. To get the benefits of turmeric, you can add it to your favorite dishes such as curries, soups, or make a warm drink called golden milk with turmeric, milk, and spices. Alternatively, you can also take turmeric supplements.

- **Ginger**

Ginger contains compounds called gingerols, which have natural anti-inflammatory and analgesic effects. You can enjoy ginger's benefits by drinking ginger tea, adding fresh ginger to your meals, or taking ginger supplements.

3. Mind-Body Techniques for Pain Management

Our minds have a great impact on how we experience and handle pain. Utilizing mind-body techniques can help us to better manage our discomfort and lessen its effect on our lives.

- **Meditation**

Meditating regularly can help alleviate pain by promoting relaxation and decreasing stress. Mindfulness meditation has been especially effective in managing pain.

- **Yoga**

Yoga is a practice that involves physical postures, breathing exercises, and meditation to help with flexibility, reduce muscle tension, and provide relief from chronic pain conditions such as lower back pain and arthritis.

- **Deep Breathing**

Taking deep breaths can help to ease tense muscles and manage pain. Try doing deep-breathing exercises when you're feeling uncomfortable or make it part of your daily routine.

- **Biofeedback**

This method can help you learn to manage your body's functions, like your heart rate and muscle tension, to lessen pain. Working with a professional can be beneficial in biofeedback sessions.

- **Visualization**

Visualization and guided imagery exercises can be useful in helping to take your mind off of pain and create a feeling of relaxation and contentment.

Incorporating natural pain relief methods into your daily routine can provide significant relief for various types of discomfort. It's important to talk to a healthcare professional, especially if you have chronic or severe pain, to make sure the remedies you choose are safe and suitable for your particular situation. In the following chapters, we'll look at more natural solutions for common health issues, giving you the power to take control of your health.

Chapter 4

Skin Care and Remedies

Maintaining healthy skin is essential for both aesthetic and health reasons. In this chapter, we'll look at natural methods and remedies that can help you achieve and keep your skin looking and feeling its best. Our skin is the largest organ of our body and also serves as our first line of defense against the outside world. Therefore, it is important to take care of it in order to maintain our overall well-being.

1. Aloe Vera for Sunburn and Skin Irritation

Aloe vera is a calming and multi-purpose plant that has been used for many years to help with a variety of skin issues. Here are some of the ways it can be beneficial for your skin:

- **Sunburn Relief**

Aloe vera gel is a great solution for sunburns. Its cooling effects can help reduce the pain, redness, and swelling that comes with too much sun. All you need to do is apply a thin layer of pure aloe vera gel to the affected area and you'll get some relief.

- **Skin Irritation**

Aloe vera is a great option for soothing minor skin issues, such as itching, rashes, and bug bites. Its anti-inflammatory and antimicrobial properties make it an ideal choice for calming inflamed skin.

2. Honey and Oatmeal Masks for Skin Rejuvenation

Honey and oatmeal are two ingredients that are commonly found in the kitchen, but they also have amazing advantages for your skin.

- **Honey**

Raw honey is an amazing natural humectant, meaning it helps keep your skin hydrated. It also has antibacterial properties that can be great for those with acne-prone skin. Applying honey as a face mask can give your skin a healthy, glowing appearance.

- **Oatmeal**

Ground oats can be a great way to slough off dead skin cells and unblock pores. An oatmeal mask can be a great way to soothe sensitive skin and reduce redness and inflammation. To get the most out of this treatment, mix oatmeal with either water or yogurt to create a calming paste that can be applied to your face for a refreshing experience.

3. Natural Solutions for Acne and Eczema

Dealing with acne and eczema can be difficult, but natural remedies can provide some relief.

- **Acne**

Tea tree oil has antimicrobial properties, so it can be diluted and used on areas of the skin that are prone to acne to help clear up blemishes. Additionally, aloe vera and honey masks can be used to soothe irritated skin and reduce inflammation caused by acne.

- **Eczema**

Coconut oil is a widely-used natural remedy for eczema. Its moisturizing qualities can help to ease dry, itchy skin. To lock in moisture, simply spread a thin layer of coconut oil on the affected areas. Taking an oatmeal bath can also be beneficial in soothing irritated skin.

It's important to be aware that everyone's skin is different and that reactions to natural remedies can vary. Before trying any new product, it's essential to do a patch test, especially if you have sensitive or allergy-prone skin. To keep your skin healthy, make sure to stay hydrated, eat a balanced diet full of antioxidants, and protect it from too much sun exposure. By following these practices, you can nurture and revitalize your skin, giving it a healthy and glowing look. In the upcoming chapters, we'll discuss more natural remedies for various health issues, helping you to adopt a holistic approach to wellbeing.

Chapter 5
Stress Management and Mental Health

In this day and age, stress is a common part of life. But how we handle it can have a major effect on our mental and emotional health. This chapter looks at natural methods and techniques that can help you find inner calm, decrease stress, and look after your mental well-being.

1. Lavender and Chamomile for Stress Relief

Lavender and Chamomile are two herbs that are well-known for their ability to help reduce stress and promote relaxation.

- **Lavender**

Lavender essential oil is renowned for its calming aroma. You can use it to create a peaceful atmosphere in your home by diffusing it, adding it to a warm bath, or applying it topically (diluted) to help you relax and reduce stress and anxiety.

- **Chamomile**

Chamomile tea is a great, natural way to reduce stress and anxiety. Its compounds have a soothing effect on the nervous system, making it an excellent choice for winding down before bed.

2. Yoga and Meditation for Mental Well-Being

Yoga and meditation are powerful practices that promote mental clarity, relaxation, and emotional balance:

- **Yoga**

Doing yoga is a combination of physical poses, breathing control, and meditation. Practicing yoga regularly can help to reduce stress, improve your mood, and boost your mental health. Additionally, it can increase your physical flexibility and strength.

- **Meditation**

Meditating can help you become more mindful and aware of yourself, which can help you better manage stress and anxiety. Even a few minutes of meditation each day can have a significant effect on your mental well-being, providing a sense of serenity and understanding. Both yoga and meditation can be tailored to fit your individual needs and desires, making them accessible to people of all ages and fitness levels.

3. The Gut-Brain Connection and Mood

Recent studies have revealed the intricate bond between the gut and the brain, referred to as the gut-brain connection. This connection has far-reaching implications for one's emotional state and mental well-being.

- **Probiotics**

Including probiotic supplements and fermented foods, such as yogurt and kefir, in your diet can help to maintain a healthy gut microbiome. A balanced gut microbiome has been linked to better mental health and a decreased risk of depression and anxiety.

- **Fiber-Rich Diet**

Eating a lot of fiber-rich foods, such as fruits, vegetables, and whole grains, can be beneficial for your gut. Fiber acts as a prebiotic, providing nourishment to the helpful bacteria in your digestive system.

- **Avoiding Gut Irritants**
Eating fewer processed foods, reducing sugar intake, and avoiding artificial additives can help keep the gut lining healthy. This is essential for proper nutrient absorption and for regulating mood.

Maintaining your gut health through diet and incorporating stress-reducing activities like yoga and meditation into your daily routine can have a positive effect on your mental health. It's important to remember that managing stress and supporting mental health is an ongoing process, and these natural remedies and practices can be useful in your journey towards finding inner peace and emotional strength.

In the upcoming chapters, we'll look at natural remedies for common health issues, so you can take a holistic approach to your wellbeing.

Chapter 6
Home Remedies for Cold and Flu

The common cold and seasonal flu are two of the most frequent illnesses we experience. Although they usually pass on their own, there are some natural remedies and practices that can help reduce symptoms, strengthen your immune system, and help you get better faster. In this chapter, we'll look at some of the best home remedies for colds and flu.

1. Elderberry Syrup and Honey-Ginger Tea

Two comforting and soothing remedies that can help ease cold and flu symptoms are elderberry syrup and honey-ginger tea. These two drinks can provide relief from the symptoms of these illnesses.

- **Elderberry Syrup**

Elderberries are full of antioxidants and have been used for centuries to help bolster the immune system. You can easily find elderberry syrup or supplements to help reduce the length and intensity of cold and flu symptoms.

- **Honey-Ginger Tea**

A cup of honey-ginger tea is a classic remedy for sore throats, coughs, and congestion. Honey has natural antibacterial properties that can help reduce throat irritation. Ginger has anti-inflammatory and warming

effects, which can help alleviate symptoms and provide relief.
 To make honey-ginger tea, just steep some fresh ginger slices in hot water, add a spoonful of honey, and enjoy.

2. Nasal Irrigation and Steam Inhalation

Having a stuffy nose and feeling pressure in your sinuses are typical signs of colds and flu. If you're looking for relief, there are two natural methods you can try: steam inhalation and nasal irrigation.

- **Nasal Irrigation**

Rinsing your nasal passages with a saline solution can help clear out mucus and reduce congestion. Neti pots and saline nasal sprays are easy to find and can be used as instructed to get some relief.

- **Steam Inhalation**

If you're feeling congested or have irritated nasal passages, try inhaling steam from a bowl of hot water. To make the remedy even more effective, add a few drops of eucalyptus or peppermint essential oil to the hot water. To use the remedy, drape a towel over your head and lean over the bowl, breathing in the steam for a few minutes.

3. Rest and Hydration for Recovery

One of the best strategies to get over a cold or flu is to give your body the rest and fluids it needs.

- **Rest**

When you're feeling under the weather, your body needs extra energy to battle the sickness. Make sure you get enough rest and let your immune system do its thing.

- **Hydration**

It's important to stay hydrated when you're sick. Drinking plenty of water, herbal teas, and clear broths can help keep your body hydrated and thin out mucus secretions, making it easier to clear congestion.

- **Nutrient-Rich Foods**

Eating nutrient-dense foods such as fruits, vegetables, and soups can give your body the vitamins and minerals it needs to heal.

- **Avoid Alcohol and Caffeine**

It's a good idea to stay away from these substances when you're feeling under the weather, as they can cause dehydration.

If you want to get over cold and flu symptoms quickly, it's important to get enough rest and stay hydrated. Additionally, you can try some home remedies to help your body recover. However, if your symptoms don't improve or get worse, it's

essential to see a doctor for proper diagnosis
and treatment.

In the upcoming chapters, we'll look at
different natural remedies to help you take
charge of your health.

Chapter 7

Natural Remedies for Allergies

Allergies can be a real nuisance, but there are ways to manage them without relying on medication. In this chapter, we'll look at some natural remedies and lifestyle changes that can help you cope with allergy symptoms.

1. Local Honey and Bee Pollen

Honey and bee pollen from local sources have become increasingly popular as natural treatments for allergies, especially those related to the changing of the seasons. *Here's how they can help to alleviate symptoms:*

- **Local Honey**

Eating a bit of honey from your local area may help your body become less sensitive to the pollen in the air. The concept is that by taking in small amounts of pollen from your environment, your immune system will become less reactive to it in the long run.

- **Bee Pollen**

Bee pollen is a nutrient-packed substance that bees collect. It has a range of vitamins, minerals, and antioxidants. Some people think that taking bee pollen supplements can help strengthen their immunity to allergens.

However, there is not much scientific evidence to back up these claims, so it is best to talk to a healthcare professional before trying them, especially if you have serious allergies.

2. Quercetin and Other Natural Antihistamines

Quercetin is a flavonoid found in many fruits and vegetables that has natural antihistamine properties. It works by inhibiting the release of histamine, which is responsible for allergic reactions. Apples, onions, citrus fruits, and leafy greens are all good sources of quercetin, and you can also find it in supplement form at health food stores.

Eating quercetin-rich foods or taking a supplement may help to reduce allergy symptoms.

Other natural antihistamines include bromelain (found in pineapple) and stinging nettle. While these are believed to have anti-allergy effects, more research is needed to understand their full benefits.

3. Reducing Allergen Exposure at Home

It is essential to reduce allergen exposure in the home in order to effectively manage allergies.

- **Dust and Mold**

Maintaining a clean and well-ventilated home is essential to reduce dust and mold allergens. To further reduce allergens, use allergen-proof covers on pillows and mattresses, and make sure to wash bedding regularly in hot water.

- **Pollen**

During peak pollen seasons, it is important to keep windows and doors closed. To help trap allergens, you should also use high-efficiency particulate air (HEPA) filters in your home's heating and cooling systems.

- **Pet Allergens**

If you have allergies to animals, it's a good idea to invest in HEPA air purifiers and make sure your pets are groomed regularly. Additionally, it's helpful to designate certain areas of your home as pet-free zones to reduce your exposure to allergens.

- **Food Allergies**

If you suffer from food allergies, it is important to be vigilant when reading food labels and to make sure to inform your server when eating out. Additionally, if you have been prescribed an epinephrine auto-injector, make sure to always have it with you.

It's important to keep in mind that everyone's allergies are different. If your symptoms are severe or persistent, it's best to talk to an allergist or healthcare provider to get a personalized plan for managing your allergies.

Taking practical steps to reduce allergen exposure, in addition to using natural remedies, can help you better cope with allergies and improve your quality of life.

Chapter 8

Holistic Wellness and Prevention

As we come to the end of our exploration of natural remedies, it is essential to stress the significance of holistic wellness and prevention. Achieving true well-being is more than just treating individual issues; it involves taking care of your body, mind, and soul to maintain a balanced and healthy lifestyle. In this last chapter, we will look at the basics of holistic wellness and how to incorporate natural remedies into your daily life for long-term health.

1. The Role of Nutrition and Whole Foods

Eating right is essential for achieving holistic wellness. What you consume has a direct impact on your physical health, energy levels, and even your emotional state. To make nutrition a priority in your holistic wellness plan, here are some tips:

- **Whole Foods**

It's important to focus on eating whole, unprocessed foods like fruits, vegetables, whole grains, lean proteins, and healthy fats. These foods are packed with essential nutrients, fiber, and antioxidants that are beneficial for your health.

- **Balanced Diet**

It is important to strive for a healthy diet that includes a variety of foods from all food groups. This way, you can ensure that you are getting a wide range of essential nutrients to keep your body functioning properly.

- **Hydration**

It is essential to stay hydrated for your body to function properly. This includes digestion, circulation, and detoxification. Make sure to drink lots of water throughout the day.

- **Mindful Eating**

Be mindful when you eat by listening to your body's signals of hunger and fullness. Taking your time to enjoy your food can help you to have a better relationship with food and aid digestion.

2. Integrating Natural Remedies into Your Daily Routine

If you want to fully embrace holistic wellness, why not try adding natural remedies into your daily routine as a way to take preventive action and look after yourself?

- **Morning Routine**

Begin your morning with a cup of herbal tea or a smoothie packed with antioxidants, such as berries and leafy greens.

- **Stress Management**

Take a few minutes each day to do something calming, such as meditating, doing yoga, or taking deep breaths.

- **Healthy Snacking**

Opt for healthy snacks like nuts, seeds, and fresh fruit to keep your energy levels steady throughout the day.

- **Regular Exercise**

Incorporate physical activity into your daily life. Take a brisk walk, go for a bike ride, or try a dance class - find something you enjoy to stay active.

- **Adequate Sleep**

Getting enough sleep is important, so make sure to set a regular bedtime and create a space that is conducive to rest.

- **Herbal Supplements**

If you discover natural remedies that are effective for you, think about adding them to your daily regimen as supplements or teas.

3. Building a Holistic Wellness Plan

To devise a thorough wellness plan, take into account the following steps:

- **Assess Your Goals**

Figuring out which aspects of your health and wellbeing you want to prioritize is important. This could include physical fitness, mental health, stress management, or getting better sleep.

- **Set Realistic Goals**

Divide your objectives into achievable, doable parts. Begin with something small and gradually increase your accomplishments.

- **Seek Professional Guidance**

It's a good idea to talk to healthcare professionals, like nutritionists, fitness trainers, or holistic practitioners, to create a wellness plan that is tailored to your individual needs and objectives.

- **Stay Consistent**

It is essential to be consistent in order to achieve long-term success. Make sure to incorporate your chosen wellness practices into your daily routine and make them an absolute necessity in your life.

- **Reflect and Adjust**

It's important to take stock of your progress and make changes as necessary. Well-being is a continuous journey, and your needs may evolve over time.

By taking a holistic approach to well-being, you can create a healthier, more fulfilling life. Don't forget that natural remedies are only one part of the equation. Combining nutrition, self-care habits, and a preventive attitude will give you the power to live your best life and experience long-term wellbeing.

Conclusion

Certainly, here is the concluding chapter of your ebook "Natural Remedies for Everyday Ailments":

- **Empowering Yourself with Natural Remedies**

On this voyage of discovery into the realm of natural remedies for everyday ailments, you have set out on a mission to empower yourself and take charge of your health in a holistic manner. You have discovered the amazing potential of nature's healing powers and how they can be used to alleviate common health issues.

It is important to remember that the capacity to heal often lies within you, and natural remedies can support your body's natural healing ability. By incorporating these remedies into your life, you are not only treating the symptoms but also nurturing your body's overall wellbeing.

- **Embracing a Balanced and Healthy Lifestyle**

Living a balanced and healthy lifestyle is the key to making natural remedies work. Along with learning about herbs, plants, and holistic treatments, it's important to remember to eat nourishing foods, exercise regularly, and manage stress. These lifestyle factors are the basis of your health and wellbeing.

By taking a holistic approach to health, you can not only prevent common illnesses, but also boost your body's ability to heal and thrive. This means that you are tackling the source of health issues, rather than just treating the symptoms.

- **Resources for Further Exploration**

Beginning your exploration of natural remedies is just the start of your journey. To further your quest for health and wellbeing, here are some helpful resources to broaden your understanding and delve into the realm of natural healing.

1. Books and Magazines
There are plenty of books and magazines devoted to herbal medicine, homeopathy, and natural remedies. Make sure to look for reliable sources written by experts in the field.

2. Online Communities
Join online forums, social media groups, or websites that focus on natural remedies. Interacting with a group of like-minded people can give you valuable information and support.

3. Holistic Health Practitioners
Think about consulting with holistic health practitioners, such as naturopathic doctors, herbalists, or traditional Chinese medicine practitioners, for personalized advice.

4. Workshops and Classes
Go to workshops and classes on herbalism, aromatherapy, and other holistic practices to expand your knowledge and practical skills.

5. Herb Gardens: Plant your own herb garden to grow medicinal plants and try out remedies yourself.

6. scientific Research
 Keep up with the latest scientific research related to natural remedies and their effectiveness in treating various health conditions.

I hope this ebook has motivated you to take advantage of the amazing world of natural remedies and embark on a journey of wellness that is in line with the knowledge of nature. May your journey be full of health, energy, and the delight of uncovering the healing power that is all around us every day.

I want to thank you for joining me on this journey and I wish you a life full of vibrant health and joy. Remember that your health is a lifelong process, and there is always more to learn. By continuing to investigate and incorporate natural remedies into your life, you are taking a proactive and empowering approach to your well-being.